CW00481774

Build Empathy in Teens

A Guidebook for Teens to Develop Social Skills, Empathy, and Boost Confidence

By

Sami Publishing

About the Author

K. Olson is a clinical psychologist turned author, who is committed to assisting teens in developing core social skills for helping them to become independent adults and lead fulfilling lives.

She has spent more than 20 years studying psychology, with an emphasis on parenting and childhood development. Ms. Olson first became aware of the challenges that teenagers encounter when she experienced her own self-confidence, self-esteem, and social anxiety challenges as a teenager. She started a career in youth mentoring because she wanted to help teenagers in overcoming similar challenges that she had to confront. Her experience of working with teenagers includes those who struggle with social anxiety and, ADHD. Her innate desire to help those in need is what motivates her to write, and she is committed to making that assistance available to everyone.

Table of Contents

Introducing a Teenager's Life

- *Have you ever felt that you have little to no empathy for other people?*
- *Are you having trouble making connections because you lack social skills?*
- *Do you wish to boost your self-confidence?*

"Peace starts with learning to put oneself in another person's position and understanding the world from their perspective, and it's up to you to bring that about. A character trait that has the power to transform the world is empathy."

Empathy is one of the most crucial social skills a teen can acquire. Understanding and sharing other people's emotions is called empathy. We all possess this ability, although some people have it considerably more than others. It is an essential skill because it can improve all human interactions. Empathy allows us to relate to people more deeply and comprehend them better. It differs from having compassion for someone, which entails having sympathy or sadness for someone after observing their suffering from the outside. The ability to experience another person's suffering or see the world from their point of view is known as empathy. It's also a precursor to compassion, which is empathy in action and a commitment to doing something to lessen another person's suffering. This book will explain how empathy functions and, more significantly, will provide you with practical guidelines for improving your empathy.

The teenage years are the most challenging phases of a person's life. Since you have been living these years, you know this is true. As a teen, I had a really poor social life. Owing to my lack of confidence, it was quite challenging for me to look someone in the eyes. I even experienced bullying from my classmates. One day, after having an emotional reflection on my life and some events that had caused me to cry, I concluded that my issue stemmed from a lack of social skills. I was not self-confident enough to defend my rights; I could not strike up a basic conversation with my peers, and I could not even tell my parents when I was being bullied. My breakthrough started when I became aware of these flaws. "*Enough is enough,*" I told myself. My life radically transformed after I started practicing and using social skills. My grades and confidence both boosted, as a result. Many teenagers of today are experiencing what I did 36 years ago, which motivated me to write this book to support teenagers currently dealing with the same problem.

Considering this book, you have taken a wise step towards developing into a self-confident, empathetic, and friendly person who can talk to everyone, speak up when something is wrong, stand up for their rights, and be who they want to be.

You know those individuals who can enter a gathering and cause everyone to gravitate around them? They are outgoing, friendly, and always have something to say to start a worthwhile conversation. Most of the teenagers I mentor, nor I, are one of those people. Yes, that's true. I help teenagers in developing self-confidence, social skills, and empathy because these qualities don't develop naturally. Instead of being a high performer with supportive parents, I had a hard time as a teen. The emotional turbulence brought on by friendship issues and social expectations were tough for me to handle. Going somewhere unfamiliar and attempting new things were something I feared doing. My biggest worry was initiating a conversation with strangers since I was never sure what to say. My emotional breakdowns were brought on by my anxiety and shame, which wounded the people I loved the most. When my older sister Natalia died in an accident, it was a wake-up call for me. The pain and sadness of losing her broke me. Simultaneously, it also made me realize that I shouldn't take my life for granted.

I realized I needed to develop emotional control and social skills, reduce my anxiety, and boost my confidence. I was able to give up the excuses and surrendered my "*victim card*" by working hard to enhance my social skills. I became a qualified life coach at the age of thirty-six to empower young people like you.

If you feel connected with these challenges, I am very glad you are reading this book. You can utilize this book as a guide to get through these challenges. Even though it might not come naturally to you to be confident in social circumstances, you can work on it to boost your self-confidence. This book will walk you through the process in detail. I'm not here to criticize you or offer you advice. As your mentor and coach, I'm here to help you become your best self. I'll share some easy techniques to help you connect with others and better manage your emotions so that you always feel more confident. You share the same anxieties, worries, and insecurities I faced as a fellow human. However, I know you can quit allowing your anxieties to keep you back, just like I did. Building those social skills requires practice, but I'm here to assist you at every turn. I believe you might be astonished by how much more you'll get out of life once you stop worrying or living in fear about what people think.

Many social skills and confidence building techniques are included in this book, which many teenagers require. The desire to interact with others is the most critical factor in acquiring these skills. The development of social skills can be significantly enhanced through conversation. With your buddies, put your skills to the test while keeping an eye on your behavior. So try to learn from it and then utilize it to initiate the conversation. You'll see there's nothing to be afraid of once you start a conversation with a stranger. Self-confidence is essential for skill development; therefore, if it's low, work on raising it. The practical methods for enhancing social skills, boosting confidence, and developing empathy are covered in this guide.

So let's get started.

Chapter 1: Empathy to the Rescue

"Empathy is the ability to perceive with another person's eyes
Hear with another person's ears,
And feel with another person's heart."

In this chapter, you will discover the benefits of empathy and learn how to be more empathetic to improve and empower your life. Empathy is like a psychological hug for others. Leaning in with compassion is what empathy entails. It is the capacity to observe a situation from another person's viewpoint rather than your own to comprehend their thoughts and feelings. It isn't about making a situation about yourself; it is about concentrating on the other person who needs that emotional connection.

1.1 Understanding Empathy

Empathy is the ability to listen, hold space, refrain from passing judgment, emotionally connect, and convey the profoundly healing idea that you are not alone. Being able to understand and feel another person's feelings is known as empathy. You might act compassionately and try to improve someone else's situation if you put yourself in their position. You can do this to lessen yours and the other person's distress. There are other things besides difficulties that require empathy. You can feel your sibling's joy when they are excited about something. You can feel your friend's amusement when they are laughing at a joke. As you connect with your friends and loved ones' thoughts and feelings, and they do the same, you can improve your relationships. Empathy can also be extended to strangers. For instance, if you noticed someone sitting alone at a social gathering, you could empathize with them and initiate a conversation. You could be inspired to donate money to help those in need if you saw photographs of people suffering on the other side of the globe.

On the other hand, you might feel more upbeat when you watch a crowd cheering on television. Their joy inspires your personal joy. Imagine a scenario where you call a friend in your time of greatest emotional need in the hopes that he can offer you some solace. Instead of listening to you and giving you words of comfort, your friend could hardly wait to finish the call before you. What would you think? Nobody would likely feel comfortable about that, in my opinion. When we have individuals in our corner who are constantly willing to listen to us and comfort us when it is necessary, we flourish as humans. Without empathy, people will find it difficult to relate to one another or consider the other person's interests, and relationships will suffer as a result.

"If you plant lettuce and it doesn't grow well, you don't blame the lettuce. You investigate the causes of its poor performance. It might require fertilizer, extra water, or less sunlight. You never assign blame to the lettuce but, when we encounter issues with our friends or family, we blame the other person. However, if we know how to care for them, they will flourish like lettuce. Trying to convince someone using reason and argument or by placing blame has no beneficial results. That has been my experience. Simply demonstrating that you understand and are capable of loving will cause the situation to change. There is no need for judgment, justification, or argument."

Types of Empathy
Now that we know what empathy is, it's time to introduce the classification of empathy. These abilities might indeed be of

various kinds depending on how they are used. So let's examine the different types of empathy.

- **Cognitive Empathy**

Understanding what another person might be thinking is referred to as cognitive empathy. It is less about the ability to put ourselves in another person's shoes because it emphasizes thinking more than emotions and feelings. Therefore, even though it does not cause us to have an emotional or effective connection with the other person, it may be quite helpful to encourage them, deal with them, and comprehend their viewpoints on a particular subject. This type of empathy focuses more on the intellectual than the dynamic.

- **Affective Empathy**

Affective or emotional empathy is defined as the capacity to put ourselves in another person's shoes. The emotions and feelings of another person become contagious things that we take in and feel as if they were our own. On an emotional and even physical level, you can experience another person's feelings. It is important to note that this type of empathy is not always beneficial. It is if we can control it because it is necessary for many aspects of our lives, but if we feel overpowered by these outside emotions, it can become detrimental to our mental health. Consequently, exercising self-control is crucial.

- **Compassionate Empathy**

Compassionate empathy motivates us to assist others if we notice that they require (or may require) our assistance. It compels us to lend a hand out of the blue and has a vital humanitarian component

- **Motor Empathy**

Motor empathy is a mechanism that originates in the subconscious and causes us to mimic the facial expressions of others unconsciously. It has more to do with a propensity to mimic another person's nonverbal cues or physical responses than processing other people's emotions and feelings.

- **Emotional Empathy**

As a subset of emotional intelligence, emotional empathy enables individuals to comprehend and relate to the emotional condition of another. Understanding the emotions and motivations of others can be accomplished with the help of emotional empathy. An illustration of emotional empathy would be when a mother who has lost a kid can understand the suffering of other parents who have also lost children. Emotional empathy has a negative side as well. For instance, it could result in excessive involvement or even the encouragement of abusive behavior in a relationship.

How Do We Feel Empathy?

According to many neuroscientists, empathy is essentially the act of reproducing the identical feelings we observe in others; *The Simulation Theory*. However, preliminary research indicates that our brains include specialized "mirror neurons" that become active when we perceive and experience emotions. Many researchers think that these mirror neurons are what develop empathy. Some scientists think that only the intellect can develop empathy. According to the theory, we can feel empathy when we see other people and have an intellectual knowledge of how we should feel or respond to their emotions.

1.2 Empathy vs. Sympathy

It's common to employ both sympathy and empathy interchangeably. Only one of these, however, allows relationships to flourish beyond the surface. So what makes empathy different from sympathy? Which should you put into practice? Let's examine the differences between empathy and sympathy and discover which one can help you connect with others more effectively in daily life.

Empathy vs. Sympathy: Key Characteristics

Knowing the distinctions between sympathy and empathy might help you to decide which is best for your situation. While empathy helps to develop a stronger bond, there are also occasions when a sympathetic reaction is more appropriate.

Here is an explanation of empathy and sympathy, along with some illustrations.

What is Empathy?

Empathy is "the ability to share another person's feelings" or "the sense of understanding and sharing another person's experiences and emotions." When someone is suffering, feeling sorry for them naturally leads to feelings of pity, which is not helpful. Empathy serves as a link between two individuals, opening up a space for sincerer compassion, understanding, and healing. By developing our empathy, we are better able to understand others' perspectives, which lead us to be more helpful naturally.

- *Feeling what another person is feeling*
- *Paying attention to what they are saying*

14

- *Not passing judgment*
- *Understanding subtleties and nonverbal cues*
- *Finding out their viewpoint*
- *Recognizing everyone's emotions*

The power to understand and connect with another person's feelings is known as empathy. Empathy allows you to hear what another person has to say without passing judgment. An empathic person can feel another person's feelings and understand their perspective. Your communication skills can be improved with the help of empathy. That's because you have the ability to listen to and comprehend the opinions of others thoroughly.

Empathy can even support cooperation during social challenges, according to studies. Additionally, empathy can lessen injustice and unethical behavior.

What is Sympathy?

"Sympathy is when you comprehend another person's suffering and feel sorrow or pity for the situation they are going through." It involves making a value judgment on another person's experience. It entails:

- *Thinking about how another person is feeling*
- *Delivering unasked counsel during a conversation*
- *Making judgments*
- *Observing only the superficial problem*
- *Concealing or ignoring your own emotions*

Contrary to empathy, showing sympathy does not imply that you share another person's emotions. Instead, you feel pity or

15

sorrow for another person. You feel sorry for someone, yet you can't relate to their situation. A superficial comprehension of another person's circumstances is all that is offered by a sympathetic attitude.

Giving unsolicited advice to the other person to help them deal with their feelings can also result in sympathy. Sympathetic people frequently pass judgment when giving this counsel. Sympathy still leaves room for judgment, unlike empathy.

Which Is Better: Empathy or Sympathy?

Being sympathetic won't help you build long-lasting relationships with other people. This is true because pity only offers superficial understanding. You are unable to observe things from another person's point of view.

Conversely, empathy enables you to put yourself in another person's position enabling you to meet their needs better.

Empathy vs. Sympathy Test Questions

Use these drills to evaluate your comprehension of the distinction between sympathy and empathy.

Pick the Right Word

Please choose the appropriate word to fit each of the following sentences.

1. I have _____ for our new classmate since I am aware of how it feels to switch schools in the middle of the school year.
2. I don't know what Erica is going through, but I definitely have _____ for her situation.

Answer Guide
Utilize the answer key below to verify your responses.
1. *Empathy*
2. *Sympathy*
3. *Sympathy*
4. *Sympathy*

1.3 Importance of Empathy

Your life will benefit greatly from empathy. Your relationships with the people you interact with can become stronger as a result. You may help people feel heard and understood by making an effort to understand them. They will consequently be more inclined to spend the time empathizing with you as well. This strengthens your bond and fosters the sense of closeness that we all yearn for. According to research, a person's happiness tends to rise when they have a robust social support system. Empathy can be crucial in creating a more fulfilling life since it improves connections. Empathy can also:

✓ **Motivate Helping Behavior**

> Your capacity for empathy may inspire you to take steps to make other people's lives better. These deeds could be as simple as giving to a good cause or simply giving someone a hug to make them feel better.

✓ **Help You Work on Your Acceptance Skills**

You can improve your ability to tolerate others by using empathy. In other words, it makes it simpler for you to develop social relationships by promoting more understanding and acceptance of others.

✓ **Helps You Establish Closer Relationships**

You can relate to someone better by trying to imagine yourself in their situation. Doing so encourages the development of closer bonds. In other words, you're not merely spending time with the individual; instead, you're attempting to understand them better. This encourages deep relationships rather than fleeting ones.

✓ **Helps You Get to Know People Better**

As you can see, empathy enables you to relate to other people. As a result, people will open up to you and be more inclined to reveal their true selves, which in turn helps you get to know them better. Additionally, getting to know individuals and forming connections with them enables you to grow yourself.

✓ **Boosts Your Self-Esteem**

Those who show empathy are more successful and collaborative, which raises their self-esteem.

1.4 The Gift of Empathy is a Blessing!!!

Even while having the ability to empathize with others might be overwhelming at times, it's unquestionably one of the greatest blessings you can possess. You are an empath if you have ever been profoundly affected by another person's emotions or if you have a keen awareness of your surroundings. When you can use your empathy to understand others, especially in circumstances where you might not otherwise be able to, being empathic can undoubtedly be a blessing. It enables you to have a closer bond with those who are essential to you, allowing you to sense their distress even when they are unable to voice it. Here are some good reasons why having the gift of empathy is a blessing.

- *Feel Other People's Emotions*

You're quite good at perceiving other people's thoughts and feelings in addition to comprehending their points of view. Furthermore, they don't even need to verbalize their feelings for you to be able to understand them. You can sometimes tell if someone is in a terrible mood or overly happy just by sharing a room with them. You will be able to identify whether someone is feeling fear, rage, or grief right away. One of the most incredible presents anyone could ever hope for is that you will always be there for your loved ones in that same spirit.

- *Helping Those in Need*

You are incredibly helpful and supportive due to your empathy gift. You naturally desire to assist your friends or family members when you find them in need but your willingness to help others is not limited to those close to you. Empaths are drawn to others who are suffering by their generosity and openness.

- *Strong Gut Feeling*

You're strong at picking up on tiny changes in tone, body language, and facial expressions because you have the ability to feel beyond words. Another factor making the ability to empathize is a strong intuition.

- **Highly Aware of the World Around You**

You are more conscious of your surroundings, making it easier to spot any threats, dangers, or negative energy. Having the ability to recognize danger and defend yourself from it is actually a spiritual gift. If you find that you suddenly feel down, your inner alarm may be sounding to warn you to avoid the situation.

- **Natural Healer**

Your presence alone can often be calming to others and has the ability to heal since you are able to empathize with and feel exactly what the other person is feeling. Your ability to empathize with people helps them feel safe, and at ease around you, which gives them the space they need to recover more rapidly just by being in your presence. Empathy is a major blessing because one of the greatest spiritual gifts is being a natural healer.

- **Understand People Better**

Empaths are better able to comprehend other individuals because they have the capacity to look under the surface. If you possess empathy, you may easily recognize another person's feelings while also understanding their viewpoint.

You have the ability to interpret a person's body language and are never quick to pass judgment. Instead, one of your greatest gifts is your patience with people.

1.5 Lack of Empathy: The Root of All Evils

You can see how lacking empathy can be harmful if you realize that empathy is crucial to how we relate to and connect with others. Here are just a few of the issues teens may encounter due to not having empathy.

❖ *Quickness to Criticize*

Lower empathy makes it more necessary to criticize others who don't live up to your standards or your beliefs of what people ought to be like. You are less likely to try to understand why someone thinks or behaves the way they do when you don't feel an emotional connection to them.

❖ *Unusual Responses to Grief*

A lack of empathy may become apparent under challenging circumstances. Someone in your life probably cannot understand your sadness if they don't seem to care or express any form of empathy when you experience grief.

For instance, if you have lost a pet that you cherished dearly, most people will feel bad for you and comprehend your pain and sense of loss. A person who lacks empathy won't get why you're unhappy and might say something hurtful.

❖ *Egotistical*

A strong sense of self accompanies a lack of empathy. A person who lacks empathy is likely to be exceedingly egotistical since they put themselves first in every circumstance. These people constantly demand attention, behave carelessly, and are unable to put themselves in another person's position. This could be applied to anything, and some instances of this behavior include pushing past people in line at the coffee shop and careless driving.

❖ **Loneliness**

Amazed? Most likely not. People who lack empathy frequently become isolated. They're not very good at establishing and maintaining long-lasting connections. Additionally, the person with no empathy can't help but notice how people are constantly leaving their social circle.

❖ **A Sense of Entitlement**

People who lack empathy frequently engage in constant self-talk. Any conversational turn that does not focus on them will be ignored. Many people can engage in this conduct, which is referred to as conversational narcissism, without actually being narcissists.

In your life, there may be a few examples of such people. Perhaps you might have a friend that is constantly requesting favors from you with no guarantee that he will return the favors. They may be simply unaware of the need to put up a similar amount of effort in the relationship and are not thinking about how their behavior can affect you.

1.6 Essential Characteristics of Empathy

Empathy encompasses more than just feelings and emotions. In order to provide compassionate, observant, and helpful support, we must also consider people's internal states and viewpoints.

Here I'll briefly define some characteristics of empathy listed by McLaren.

- **Emotional Contagion**

  Being able to sense and recognize other people's emotions is referred to as emotional contagion. There is much more to empathy than just this essential characteristic. Some of us merely possess that, and some of us are so empathic that the emotions of others completely overcome us. If other people's feelings completely take us over, we won't be able to respond to others' emotions with empathy. However, an important characteristic is an emotional contagion, the capacity to sense other people's emotions or to identify those emotions through nonverbal cues, signals, and other means.

- **Perspective-Taking**

  This ability enables you to creatively put yourself in other people's shoes, view things from their perspective, and precisely perceive what they could be feeling. This helps you grasp what other people might desire or need.

- **Perceptive Engagement**

  The capacity to respond effectively to address the needs of others is referred to as perceptive engagement. We must possess this ability to discern what other people need and feel.

- **Empathic Accuracy**

  This is your capacity to recognize and accurately comprehend the emotional states and intentions of both yourself and others.

1.7 My Own Story!!!

My mother and I don't get along very well. I've been "working" on my connection with my father for the last 20 years as I try to

23

figure out how to forgive him for abusing me as a child while he was an alcoholic. Although it is not simple, I keep trying and pushing through. My mother asked me to organize a party for my Dad's 80th birthday on Father's Day. In order to facilitate my recovery, I had my concerns about celebrating his eighty years of life in the presence of relatives I had become distant from them over time but my empathy compelled me to get in touch with my brother, organize an event, and celebrate my Dad's eight-decade journey. Why? Because it wasn't about me. I envisioned how it would be for my parents, and I tried to understand their emotions. Not for my comfort but rather because I could feel the hurt, remorse, and apology in my parents' hearts for being unsatisfactory parents. The birthday celebration was ultimately worthwhile. I have no regrets about the expression in Father's elderly eyes as we all surprised him. Empathy compels us to help others, even when it is uncomfortable for us. We persevere after realizing how others are feeling. We are sensitive to the discomfort and sadness of others, but we also absorb their joy and internalize it.

1.8 Living Examples of Empathy

Everyone agrees that empathy is crucial, yet sometimes it can be challenging to spot it in action. These living instances of empathy will aid you in recognizing scenarios where it is appropriate to demonstrate empathy.

⭐ A Friend Fails a Test

Imagine you are a student whose classmate has recently failed a significant test or exam. Your friend is upset because, despite her best efforts, she failed to pass her class. Even if you did well on this test, you know what failure feels like. You don't attempt to make things better for your pal. Instead, you say something empathetic like, *"I apologize sincerely about your grade. I know how diligently you studied and how discouraged you must be feeling."*

✢ A Student Gets Bullied

One student experiences bullying and stall-pushing from other students in the school restroom. Consider that you are a child witnessing this conversation. How can you show empathy? You first recall what it was like to be teased. You may wait for the bullies to leave before assisting the child out of the stall. You could also take action by telling an adult about the bullying and demonstrating compassionate empathy

✢ Putting an Animal to Sleep

People are capable of feeling empathy for other creatures. Think about your favorite dog passing away. You strive to keep her content and comfortable for as long as you can, but eventually, her pain becomes too much for her to enjoy life. You take her to the veterinarian and arrange for her death. This decision was made with empathy in mind.

1.9 Ideas to be More Compassionate towards Others

More compassionate people are needed to make the world a happier and more peaceful place to live. We must be more compassionate to end Earth's hatred, injustice, and bloodshed. Therefore, the following suggestions will assist us in developing compassion for others:

25

- ## Be Selfless

Consider others' perspectives. Put your happiness in other people's happiness. Start thinking about and caring about others instead of just yourself. Get rid of selfishness. The journey of compassion is a beautiful way to start caring for, assisting, and cheering up other people. Being selfless is a terrific way to start on the path to becoming more compassionate.

- ## Be Humble

Get rid of your pride. Stop thinking yourself better than others; stop acting as though you are an expert, own up to your mistakes, and forgive others. If you have humility in your heart, it will be simpler for you to have compassion for others because humility allows you to listen, feel, and look clearly into the hearts of others.

- ## Listen Carefully

Never turn away from someone who is speaking to you. Give them the chance to express themselves without talking too much. Learn about their experiences by hearing their stories. Recognize the points they are trying to make. Be conscious that awareness, not ignorance, is what compassion is all about.

- ## Forgive Them

When someone wrongs you, resist the need to seek retaliation. Even though your heart may be broken, you have the power to allow it to mend. You can let your heart heal by forgiving those who hurt you. Especially if they honestly plead for your forgiveness, pardon them. Recognize that they are suffering because they are also feeling sorry and guilty.

- **Do Not Judge Others**

Quit passing judgment on other people. Find something positive in others rather than focusing on their defects. Find out how you may assist them rather than pointing out their inadequacies. The goal of compassion is to uplift and support others rather than to judge and denigrate them.

- **Feel their pain**

All of us experience pain but addressing others' suffering and our own requires compassion for others. Feel your friends' suffering and offer to help them if you wish to be compassionate to them. Ensure their comfort when they experience illness, the loss of a loved one, depression due to a significant failure, or broken hearts.

1.10 Practicing Empathy in Your Daily Life

Even in animals, empathy is a fundamental element. However, a variety of factors can affect a person's ability to feel empathy, either negatively or favorably. A person's overall capacity for empathy typically remains constant throughout their lifetime.

Finding more opportunities to show empathy in your daily life is never wrong. Some excellent starting points are:

- **Listen, but Also Help**

Being empathetic toward others is only one aspect of empathy; another is demonstrating our humanity to others. Building a strong and compassionate relationship with someone else requires confidence in them to hear and understand their genuine thoughts and feelings because empathy is a two-way street.

For instance, try to learn more about the homeless person's life instead of merely passing them by in the railway station and noticing how dirty they are. This can range from simply saying hello and bringing them a food or care box to helping at a homeless shelter. Immersion in the lives and situations of others is a terrific method to develop empathy in any case.

- **Challenge Yourself**

Take on challenging tasks that require you to step outside of your comfort zone. Learn a new skill, like how to play a musical instrument, a new hobby, or a foreign language, for instance. Create a new professional skill. You will become humbler if you act this way because humility is a crucial enabler of empathy.

- **Try Perspective-Taking**

It is common to think of perspective-taking as the "precursor" of empathic concern. Increasing empathy levels and taking the first step toward becoming empathetic depend on understanding another person's perspective.

Consider other people's perspectives when appropriate, and show respect for them. It serves as a healthy exercise and prevents us from passing judgment.

- **Be Open to Changing Your Attitudes and Beliefs**

It will be quite challenging to build empathy if you are someone who is always sure that your opinions are correct all the time. It's especially crucial to change that thinking first. Be open to modifying your views and beliefs and avoid making assumptions about other people.

Chapter 2: Developing Your Empathy Skills

This chapter will discuss ideas about developing or increasing your empathy skills. One of the most significant abilities you may develop is the ability for empathy. Empathy can be a balm to fear and fury in a world that spends so much time pointing out imperfections and provoking people's wrath and fear. Empathy can make your life more satisfying and healthier for you and others. For you to be able to assist someone, you must empathize with them, put yourself in their situation, and be conscious of and sensitive to their emotions.

2.1 Walk a Mile in Someone Else's Shoes

Now, if you reflect on the past two weeks' events, I'm very sure that at least one individual has irritated you for whatever reason. If you think back on what transpired in this instance, angered feelings may flare up; however, this time, try to remember the situation as objectively as you can. You can take a moment to consider your point of view, your argument, and the motivations behind YOUR actions. Then, attempt to put yourself in the position of your opposite, the person who so greatly enraged you. Even though it could be challenging at first, try your hardest to put yourself in the other person's shoes and consider the situation from their point of view for a few moments. No matter how arrogant, irrational, or full of himself you think your opponent is, try to set your opinion of them aside for a bit. It will hopefully be possible to recognize and comprehend the motivations behind your opponent's behavior while in this state of objectivity; whether you agree with their actions or not is less crucial. Understanding the causes of your counterpart's behavior has helped you to overcome a significant obstacle on the road to compassion.

2.2 Developing Empathy Out of a Person's Motive

In addition to attempting to grasp the reasons behind someone's actions, you should also make an effort to comprehend what it would be like to be that person. From that point on, when you just partially understand the struggles and emotions the other person is going through, it will be simpler for you to empathize with them.

2.3 Replace Anger with Compassion

You can try to apply this technique to your daily tasks if you've mastered the skill of placing yourself in another person's shoes. Set a goal for yourself to respond with empathy rather than rage. By doing this, you can avoid making rapid judgments and rash actions that you may later regret.

2.4 Discover the Similarities, Not the Differences

Many people in this selfish world seem to have lost sight of the fact that everyone else is also trying to find happiness. Naturally, this will lead to conflicts because we tend to forget about others when we are focused solely on ourselves, which makes us perceive more differences between "us" and "them," even though we are all the same. Despite our moral convictions, skin tone, or religious beliefs, we all want serenity and love. Additionally, we all make our best effort to prevent misery and pain. In order to avoid being blinded by the differences that seem to set you apart from this individual, try to see your similarities with them.

2.5 Don't Judge Too Hastily

When we first meet someone, we automatically categorize them. Until we actually get to know someone better, our first impressions of them might have a lasting impact on how we see them. We frequently don't even consider this process as it takes place; instead, we rely on our "intuition" to lead us when forming judgments about other people. It is crucial that you know that this is a normal process unfolding, but regrettably, it causes many biases. It's essential to put aside your prejudices and generalizations in order to see beyond the surface when trying to empathize with others.

Before passing judgment on someone, consider whether you truly know them and are aware of the circumstances that led to their current state. You can establish an unbiased judgment about someone if you can relate to them, comprehend what they are going through on a daily basis, and acknowledge what it must feel like to be in their shoes. Nevertheless, it should be mentioned that until you have been in the same situation as another person, with the same loads, troubles, and sufferings, you should consider whether you are qualified to judge or criticize this individual. It's essential to recognize that other people also view the world through biases, values, and generalizations, which may significantly impact how they behave.

2.6 Become Aware of Your Emotional Landscape

The capability to thoroughly identify and comprehend one's own sentiments is a significant factor in determining one's ability to empathize with others. Many people struggle with this issue as they try their best to block out unwanted emotions by engaging in activities like work, watching TV, using drugs and alcohol, or engaging in other addictive behaviors. As a result, keeping a log of the various emotions we experience on a daily basis can be incredibly helpful in determining the depth of our emotional patterns. This is known as an "emotions protocol." This helps us to see that each person's emotional landscape is unique and encourages us to explore the range of our own feelings and those of others.

Write down each emotion or feeling you encountered throughout the day in five minutes to create an "emotions protocol," which doesn't take much time or effort.

2.7 Ask Others About their Perspective

You can ask people what they think about a particular circumstance or situation or how they feel about it. In this approach, you can compare your impressions with a statement rather than relying solely on your sensitivities. You are free to use this strategy anywhere you see fit. As a final point, let me say that empathy is a skill that can be learned and improved with regular practice. It is, therefore, never too late to learn it if you want to improve your comprehension of how others behave.

Chapter 3 Social Skills: You Weren't Born to Be Alone

Through this chapter, you will know what social skills are and the significance of learning them. Additionally, you'll discover some key strategies for developing social skills. Social skills are essential for teens to possess 'empathy' which can be defined as the ability to put themselves in the position of another person and identify the emotions that they are experiencing, as this enables them to respond to the emotions that others are experiencing in a manner that is compassionate and understanding.

3.1 Social Skills: What are They?

The ability to relate to people healthily and have productive relationships with them is known as social skills. This covers the communication, posture, and body language utilized in social situations. The primary goal of social skills is to enable people to engage with one another in a social setting. Through more effective communication, social skills aid in the development of better relationships. Since it makes a person a better communicator, having high social skills is favorable to social interactions and social functioning. Understanding what is appropriate and socially acceptable at different times is a necessary social ability. Humans are sociable creatures by nature. The capacity to adapt, improvise, and deal successfully in social situations can be referred to as social skills. Success in various areas, including education, and daily life, depends on one's ability to interact with others.

Not all people are born with good social skills. While some people may have a natural gift for building relationships, social skills can be learned and developed like any other ability by the others. Such skills require practice and a lot of trial and error to master.

Strong social skills are a prerequisite for having a positive impact on others. Teens with social skills can get along with people and put them at ease in various situations. Good social skills include, for example:

- *Listening intently to what is being said.*
- *Being on time.*
- *Avoiding spreading rumors about other people.*
- *Showing compassion.*
- *Posing inquiries to discover more about people.*
- *Demonstrating patience.*

Someone with low social skills is more likely to react negatively or inappropriately to others. Others can feel uneasy because of this.

Poor social skills include:

- *Being extremely pleasant when it isn't always suitable (for example, complimenting someone's attractiveness excessively).*
- *Exhibiting poor body language and eye contact.*
- *An improper or inadequate reaction to criticism or insult.*
- *Rushing to talk without allowing the other person to do so.*
- *Failing to decline requests in a respectful manner.*

Social Skills Development

For teens, social skill development is crucial to growth and development. As teens learn to connect with others, social skills start to develop. The development of social skills occurs at various stages of life and is influenced by several variables. A youngster who participates in various social activities is more likely to be socially adept than a child who stays at home all the time. Children can learn social skills in a variety of methods, including:

> ✓ *Being Asked to Express Verbally Rather than Physically*
> *Children trained to express their emotions verbally often grow more socially skilled. For instance, a youngster can avoid getting in trouble at school by learning to express anger verbally rather than acting out by bullying a classmate. This way, he can demonstrate maturity and a grasp of proper conduct.*
> ✓ *Modeling*
> *Children can learn social skills by observing how adults act in certain situations. Children pick up on appropriate behavior by observing adults using it.*
> ✓ *Praise*
> *Children who exhibit good social skills need encouragement from others to keep doing what they are doing well.*

Types of Social Skills

Social skills come in many different forms. Here are a few instances:

- **Basic Social Skills**

The first skills people learn are basic social skills essential for initiating and maintaining a conversation. Some examples of these abilities are knowing how to begin, carry on, and terminate a conversation as well as how to ask questions.

- **Effective Communication**

Effective communicators can communicate with anyone and persuade them of their point of view. They can articulate their ideas clearly, listen to what the other person has to say, and consider it.

- **Conflict Resolution**

Solving a dispute peacefully is a key component of conflict resolution. This involves being able to address the problem, identify the underlying reason, and come up with a consensus-based solution.

Importance of Social Skills

The school years are the time when a person begins to develop social skills, which are crucial for life in general. Thus, we must emphasize and praise the value of social skills for kids. People claim that no two people are alike in terms of personality. While some people are extroverted and outgoing, others may be more self-contained and prefer to engage with people less. However, the adage *"A man is a social animal"* illustrates that people must connect with one another and adhere to certain established social norms. Social skills, on the other hand, cannot be studied like other disciplines but must instead be ingrained and grown over time.

❖ To Live a Better Life, Social Skills are Essential

The general level of social skills has a direct impact on life quality. Every person aspires to have a good quality of life or to have a successful life and be content. Relationships and a means of subsistence are the two basic building blocks of human civilization, and our social skills significantly influence both.

❖ Developing Lasting Connections Requires Social Skills

Teens with social skill problems frequently have difficulty while making friends, are often lonely, and risk rejection from their peers. Since being able to communicate effectively with our peers is essential for making friends, social skills are quite crucial.

Well, it might be discovered in the early years of life, like, in the classroom, when you can overhear children utter the saddest things about how nobody likes them, they usually suffer from a lack of social skills, which is why they don't have any friends.

❖ Education Achievement Depends on Social Skills

Social competency is one of the essential factors in determining someone's future success. It means that if you examine students' grades and try to predict which ones would be able to move on, enroll in college, find employment, or create a fantastic living, unexpectedly, you would discover that the kids who are good at social skills are more likely to be able to do that.

3.2 A Bouquet of Benefits

The development of social skills aids in preparing young people for success in their transition to adulthood. Learning social skills enhances teens' interactions with peers and adults, fosters cooperative collaborations, and assists them in being helpful, considerate, and responsible members of their communities. In addition, it instills in them the ability to define and achieve personal objectives and perseverance — skills critical to their smooth transition into maturity and other aspects of life. Having strong social skills has a number of benefits. Here are some:

- **More and Better Relationships**

Being able to relate to people easily results in more incredible connections and, occasionally, outstanding friendships. Your social abilities will help you to become more charismatic, which is desirable. People are more drawn to charismatic individuals.

Most people know that solid interpersonal interactions are essential for success. You will meet new people if you put your attention on relationships. Well-developed social skills can improve your outlook on life and raise your happiness and fulfillment.

- **Better Communication**

Communication skills are naturally developed through

interpersonal interaction because effective communication is a prerequisite for having strong social skills; it is possible that mastering this ability will be your most valuable life skill.

- **Greater Efficiency**

If you have good public dealing skills, you will be able to avoid situations where you are among people you don't like as much. Some people avoid social situations because they don't want to hang out with people who don't share their interests or worldviews. *For example, attending a party will be easier for you if you know at least some of the guests.*

A robust set of social skills will enable you to gently express that you need to spend time with other people at the gathering if you are in a social scenario and do not want to spend time with "John" because you dislike him.

- **Social Relationships May Boost Mental Health**

Both extroverts and introverts benefit from feeling a sense of belonging, support, and concern from other people, which helps them both succeed. People tend to have higher self-esteem and a stronger sense of purpose when they feel supported, which may lower their risk of developing depressive and anxiety disorders.

- **Social Skills Brings Confidence**

Social skills and self-confidence go hand in hand quite well. Being surrounded by supportive people and the people you love quickly boosts your confidence, and this feeling is reflected in your day-to-day interactions. This confidence then motivates us to keep making new connections, fostering new relationships, and preserving existing ones.

- **You Can Explore Different Cultures**

You probably will encounter a lot of individuals over time from various cultures and foreign nations if you are sociable and enjoy interacting with others. They will also give you a deep understanding of their local cultures if you hang out with them frequently and grow to be good friends. They may even take you with them when they visit their families in their home country.

Therefore, social skills can also be very beneficial for you in this regard if you are truly interested in discovering new cultures, learning about new social norms, and broadening your cultural knowledge.

- **Socializing Can Expand Your Horizon**

Another advantage of social skills is that they can broaden your perspective and help you comprehend how the world actually operates. In fact, if you spend all of your time alone at home, you'll frequently find yourself isolated and unable to appreciate how varied and fascinating life may be.

Therefore, by stepping outside of your comfort zone and meeting new people, you can also learn about various lifestyles and increase your empathy for and acceptance of others.

- **You Will Not Feel Lonely**

A lot of people can't be alone and need to be with other people all the time. Even a short period of time without the companionship of others might make some people feel rather lonely.

Therefore, practicing social skills is a terrific approach to meeting new people so that you always have someone around you if you're one of those who just can't stand being alone.

- **Makes Life Easier in General**

In one line, *"It makes our life a lot easier,"* is how I would sum up the advantages of social skills. We cannot handle all of our issues alone, but by connecting with others through social interactions, we can increase our chances of receiving assistance down the road.

3.3 Important Social Skills that Teens Need to Learn

Teens need to develop a variety of social skills in order to communicate with others and comprehend emotions in everyday situations. Additionally, it entails enhancing a teenager's linguistic skills for richer social and emotional development.

These abilities may enable teens to develop into social butterflies. If not that, then at least some social and emotional independence as they mature. Every child's social & personal needs are met when they are able to express themselves effectively. It is the most direct way to meet new people, form friendships, resolve disputes, express desires, and much more. In essence, it enables a teen to recognize social cues and effectively react to them. Like your core muscles, a strong set of social skills must constantly be developed. Many teenagers struggle with them; hence, it's crucial to understand some of the key social skills and practice them in our daily lives. The ability to interact with others is something that must be taught to our children. Don't let your teen miss out on learning these crucial social skills; teach them to your child before you send them out into the world. Here are some social skills that every teen needs to learn.

- **Learn to Read People Beyond Words**

  You must treat each individual with interest and comprehend everything they say on a deeper level than just the words they use if you want to be great at social interactions. How specifically can you accomplish this?

  Always go into conversations with the mentality that you know nothing about the other person. This is a useful skill to have if you want to comprehend people on a deeper level. It enables you to always be interested in the other person and automatically improves your listening skills. It makes you focus more intently. If you treat each individual you come into contact with as a mystery, your mind will constantly be alert and attentive to everything they are saying. You discover the meaning behind the words they say, not simply the words themselves. *What is the purpose of the narrative? What makes it so crucial? How do they feel as a result of this memory?*

  You will be able to respond to others more effectively if you can do this when speaking or listening to them. You don't only hear words; you also comprehend the feelings they convey.

- **Empathy: Understanding Other's Emotions**

You can grasp someone's emotions if you can comprehend them beyond what they say. Putting yourself in another person's shoes is a sign of empathy. You will be able to connect and comprehend others on a deeper level if you have the ability to empathize with them. If you want to be socially involved, this is a highly crucial ability to possess. Emotional intelligence is critical to utilizing your empathy abilities in social situations. Any discussion can be enjoyable for both parties if you have emotional intelligence.

The social skill of empathy is incredibly effective. When speaking to another person, you must be aware of their feelings. Which feelings are they currently experiencing? The things they say and the way they respond to you will be influenced by their emotions. If you are aware of how people feel, you must also be aware of how they desire to feel. They are most prone to react badly to a negative comment if they are feeling down. As a result, you should steer your interactions toward more uplifting topics.

You should also take into account how YOU are feeling in addition to how they are feeling. You should certainly avoid social situations altogether if you're not in the mood to talk to others. Additionally, you must be content and upbeat when conversing with others because this will influence how you act and, in turn, how others see you.

44

- **Blend in with Others**

  You should be able to blend in, which is a terrific social skill. If you can blend in, you can easily fit in with any social group, and they will be delighted to have you.

  Every time you interact with someone, be thankful. Consider it a chance to develop and make wonderful friendships. You will have a better chance of naturally integrating into any social group if you do this. Your perspective and feelings will have an impact on your actions and thoughts. If you're glad to be there, your actions and words will show it. People will be more drawn to you once they are aware of that. Blending in and being a part of other social circles will come naturally and easily if you are a source of positivity.

- **Make Social Interactions More Valuable**

  Every social encounter needs to be given consideration. To be viewed as a contributor in every social circle you join, you must actively look for ways to contribute value to those interactions. At every gathering, you need to be a source of inspiration. Make people laugh, encourage them to tell you their tales, listen to them while they do so, and make them feel valued and wanted during the engagement. Everyone will be positive around you if you express pleasant feelings.

  Give someone sound advice if they ask for it. If necessary, crack a few jokes to lighten the atmosphere. Not all circumstances need to be treated seriously. Everyone will be glad to have you around if you do this.

- **Introduce People to One Another and Aid in their Mutual Understanding**

Introducing others to one another is a fantastic approach to improving your social abilities. People will perceive you as someone who appreciates friendship if you do this. In addition to wanting to meet people, you are deemed as someone open to facilitating interactions with others. They'll even begin to give you credit for their friendship. They'll respect you more as a friend because you gave them the opportunity to become pals.

Additionally, you can introduce someone to a certain social group. Adding value to social interactions also includes introducing people to one another and fostering friendships.

Finding people with something in common is a terrific way to introduce two people. It might be something like their shared hometown, a pastime, or even just a friend. Don't forget to mention them by name as well!

You may say, *"Hey Henry, this is Mary,"* to begin the conversation. *She spent a few years residing in Minnesota. Didn't you reside there as well?* Or *"Hi Henry, this is Mary,* one of my friends. We were discussing last night's match. She just loves basketball so much, maybe even more than you do!

By doing this, you've already pointed out what the two of them have in common, and they are already familiar with one another's names before they have even spoken. This enables them to naturally continue the conversation while still being present and facilitating a smooth exchange.

- **Show Vulnerability – *It's a Social Skill!***

To make friends, you don't have to be the most exceptional person alive. Allow yourself to show humanity occasionally so that other people will know you are at ease with them. Sharing disappointing tales or even revealing a few personal secrets can help you to achieve this. You will be able to connect and comprehend others on a deeper level if you have the ability to empathize with them. Share a personal story with them when you are speaking one-on-one or in a group. Share something you've never told them before rather than revealing your deepest, most intimate secret. You are demonstrating to them your faith in them by displaying a small amount of vulnerability. They might even pay it forward by divulging some of their own secrets and stories.

As previously stated, hold off on sharing your deepest, most private secrets or experiences. It might be something foolish. However, your friends will respect you more if you admit a few of your flaws to them.

- **Build Trust with Potential Friends**

Some people lack the same level of trust as others. Many people have had situations in the past that have increased their distrust of others and increased their prudence. They are hoping to find someone they can trust. You must earn that trust by being someone deserving of it.

You might begin modestly, gradually, and steadily by revealing a few of your personal details to that person. They will feel more at ease opening up to you if you are honest with them. Slowly but consistently practice this. You two will eventually start to trust one another after sharing enough information with one another. They'll start to believe you.

- **Help Others Talk More**

You need to give other people the room to develop while you're around if you want to make friends naturally and improve your social abilities. If someone is hesitant to talk in front of people, let them speak and encourage them to do so. Being a terrific conversationalist and active listener will help you in achieving this. By exclaiming, *"that's interesting!" or "uh-huh!* You are motivating them to speak up more by occasionally saying, *"Tell me more."* Additionally, keep in mind to nod and stare at the individual while performing this.

Allowing others to share their knowledge with you is a fantastic way to aid in communication. Say something like, *"Oh, I've heard of that,"* if someone discusses their area of expertise. *"What I know about it is as follows"* ... and after you've finished, say something like, *"That's what I think. However, what do you think?"*

Just be sure that what you say about their expertise is accurate. They'll be amazed by your expertise in their subject. You are letting them instruct you by doing this. They are being given the opportunity to speak up and impart their wisdom. They will appreciate you for helping them feel better about themselves as a result of this. Just be sure to convey to them that flaws are acceptable. Tell them that you won't criticize them for their weaknesses and that having them is okay. They'll be content with opening up to you first, as your bond develops.

- **Be Friendly to Promote Warm Social Interactions**

Finally, you need to be friendly so that people can approach you. Be upbeat and joyful, and allow people to share your feelings. You must be able to engage in stimulating conversations and exhibit responsiveness if you want people to regard you as *"warm."*

Always respond to greetings with a positive statement, such as *"It's nice to meet you"* or *"I'm delighted to be here."* Tell them how appreciative you are to have their company. This should also be shown in your body language and facial gestures. Saying *"I'm pleased to be here"* should be accompanied by a grin and a solid handshake. Your body language will easily express your happiness if it is something you genuinely feel. The world appreciates a charming person, and you can be charming in this way. In front of a mirror, practice making different facial expressions. If you're unprepared, this is an excellent approach to getting ready for social situations.

Aim to convey yourself in a "natural" and not "exaggerated" manner.

If you have any unfavorable opinions, hold them to yourself unless the situation calls for it or you're with close pals. When chatting to someone you recently met, try not to let your negative feelings get the better of you. Again, smile and express gratitude for the chance. You should be thankful that you have the opportunity to create a new buddy. When you exude warmth, you can stand out from the throng right away. In general, people will look forward to meeting you, and you will automatically make a lot of friends.

3.4 Poor Social Skills Affecting Your Life

You value your social life and want it to be as fulfilling as it can be. Unfortunately, it can be challenging to build relationships or maintain the ones you already have if you exhibit some poor social skills. Poor social skills can be challenging to recognize and even more challenging to improve. It's time to improve your social skills, even if you are unaware of them, and they negatively impact your life. Some of the most typical instances of bad social skills that might harm your social life are:

- **Poor Body Language**

    Although you can't completely control your body language, you can make sure that you're conscious of your movements and how they appear to others. Avoid making any negative hand motions or gestures that could be interpreted as impolite or combative.

- **Poor Vocal Tone**

  Vocal tone describes how we communicate and how our speech sounds. Your social interactions could suffer if you have a poor vocal tone since you might come across as aggressive or furious when you're not trying to be. As a result, it's crucial to practice speaking in a polite manner.

- **Not Smiling Enough**

  In terms of communication, a smile is your most effective weapon. It can put others at ease right away and give you a friendlier appearance. Additionally, it can increase your self-esteem and confidence.

  Another effective approach to making others feel at ease around you is by smiling. So start grinning more often if you want to be more socially successful.

- **Awkward Gestures/Movements**

  We frequently make odd gestures or movements when we're anxious or uneasy, making us appear foolish and conveying the wrong messages about our personalities. Simple awkward movements include excessively rubbing your hands when you are anxious or wiping your nose when you don't have a cold.

- **Always Expecting the Other Person to Greet You First**

  People frequently make this error because they don't want to come across as desperate or in need of other people's attention. Instead of making people feel welcomed into your life when meeting new individuals for the first time,

51

this gives them the impression that they are invading your personal time and space.

- **Wanting to be Liked by Everyone**

One example of bad social skills is always trying to win people over. If someone is not interested in you, don't force them to engage in conversation with you or shake hands when you greet them. Let them take the initiative instead, and remember that being pleasant is preferable to being overly aggressive.

- **Uncomfortable Silences**

Uncomfortable silence is one of the most obvious indications that someone lacks social skills. It can be embarrassing for everyone involved when you're chatting with someone and there is an awkward silence. Let the other person speak until they have finished what they want to say if you are unsure what to say next or how to respond.

- **Being a Poor Listener**

Understanding someone's feelings about what they have said is part of understanding and simply hearing what they have to say. It's challenging for someone to open up to you and be around you if you don't comprehend how they feel about a particular subject. Therefore, if people say that you don't listen well, this may signify that your social skills need to be developed.

3.5 Habits to Win the Social Game

Our habits heavily influence our daily routine, and these simple habits significantly impact our social abilities in our social circles. However, these habits also improved my social skills to the point where people who meet me for the first time mistake me for a social butterfly. Their primary advantage, in my opinion, is that you can use half of them without anyone else's help. You can engage in those habits in the privacy of your own thoughts. Let's discuss some easy habits that will quickly get you from 0 to 100 regarding social skills.

I. React

We occasionally come across individuals who just seem strange. The conversation seems strange and unsettling, even if they respond to your questions appropriately when you speak to them. Most frequently, it happens because the other person doesn't react to what you express. Speaking to someone who doesn't react to you verbally or nonverbally is similar to talking to a wall. You can't read them, and you're unsure whether they're listening or understanding what you're saying. Reacting verbally or with your body language is the soundtrack to a discussion; without it, the scene still works, but it seems strangely barren and disjointed. Keep in mind that speaking and listening are necessary for a conversation.

II. Listen with Your Body

Learn a few essential habits that show you are paying attention to the other person. Lean toward them. Attempt to focus your attention on their face. Move your head subtly to show that you always pay attention to them.

III. Praise

Everyone enjoys receiving compliments. I've never experienced a stranger's rejection after praising them. I've never been told to "Get lost!" after complimenting someone. Although there are various responses, they all fall within the positive range. Consider the stranger and consider what you may compliment about them: their appearance, their attire, a cool tattoo, or perhaps certain conduct. It's much simpler to start a conversation with praise than to discuss life's purpose.

IV. Smile

Utilizing your smile is the next crucial element in developing social skills. Often, we are so mired in our anxieties and concerns about other people that we fail to recognize their struggles. We all feel so alone in our fast-paced environment, and a simple smile can break through those walls.

3.6 Strategies to Improve and Build Social Skills

Building strong friendships and having fun in public depends on strong social skills. You could find it difficult to talk to strangers if you believe yourself to be shy. You can profit from social skill improvement in every aspect of your life. Social skills are crucial since they can improve the effectiveness and efficiency of your communication. You can create, maintain, and nurture more meaningful relationships.

However, you may start improving your social abilities by implementing these techniques, and before long, you'll be able to start conversations confidently.

- **Behave Like a Social Person**

  You can act more socially even if you don't like being social. Don't let your fear keep you back. Regardless of nervousness, decide to talk to new individuals and engage in conversation. It will become simpler with time, and your social abilities will advance swiftly.

- **Compliment Someone**

  Giving compliments to strangers is a terrific approach to starting a conversation. Verify that they aren't rushing or preoccupied with taking a quick look at them. Then introduce yourself and provide a compliment. Share brief insights and ask questions to keep the conversation going. You can quickly improve your social skills by striking up a polite chat with a total stranger.

- **Join a Class or Club**

  An excellent place to find like-minded people is through clubs, classes, and teams. Start a discussion with a person seated next to you; if you get along well, you just might become friends! Your social skills will benefit greatly from being practiced in a lively and social setting.

- **Commit Names to Memory**

  The basis of social skills is social connections. Remember someone's name once they introduce themselves whenever you meet someone new. Ask them to repeat themselves if you can't remember right away. In a conversation, calling people by their names is a terrific way to stand out.

- **Choose General Conversation Topics**

  Great conversations are possible on broad subjects. Discuss something universal, like the weather, or comment on what is happening in your immediate surroundings rather than trying to strike up an unpleasant conversation. Maintaining a positive attitude and flowing with the flow are essential components of having effective social skills.

- **Talk About Positive Things**

  Complaining and being negative in conversation can be quite off-putting. Choose uplifting and positive themes rather than whining or making negative remarks to make a better impression. A surefire method to leave a positive impression on those around you are to be positive.

- **Leaning Forward and Keeping Your Head Up Will Help You Appear Attentive**

  You can appear interested and engaged by maintaining good posture. Cross your arms so that you appear kind and approachable during the talk. Avoid slumping or lowering your head; when you stand up straight, you seem interested in what the other person is saying. Therefore, proper posture is a fantastic method to improve your social abilities.

- **Speak Confidently in a Group**

  While in a conversation, look for opportunities to speak. Continue listening for a chance to join the conversation as it progresses. Talk confidently and boldly so that others will halt and pay attention to you.

- **End Conversations Gracefully**

  It's okay if you run out of things to say. Tell them you have to go because you have something else to do and that is all. Inform them that you appreciate their time and want to speak with them again soon. Contrary to popular belief, appropriately concluding a conversation is equally as crucial as beginning or continuing one.

- **Practice Standing Up for Yourself**

  Being outspoken does not imply selfishness or social awkwardness. It's acceptable to hold your views and opinions! Practice standing up straight and stating "no" with confidence. Ask a buddy if you can practice speaking assertively to them if you have trouble building your confidence.

- **Read Books About Social Skills**

  You can acquire specific social skills and how to strike up conversations from various publications available in the marketplaces. Though reading about these abilities won't make you an expert, keep that in mind. You'll need to practice them repeatedly.

Chapter 4: The Art of Being Confident

This chapter will teach you the value of confidence, where it originates from, and most importantly — that you are entirely capable of developing it. It will also offer tips on how to boost your self-confidence. An attitude regarding your skills and abilities is called self-confidence. It indicates that you feel in charge of your life and accept and trust yourself. Your opinion of yourself is reasonable, and you know your talents and weaknesses. You can handle criticism, speak firmly, and set reasonable goals and expectations.

On the other hand, poor self-confidence might make you feel insecure, make you docile or weak, or make it difficult for you to trust other people. You could be sensitive to criticism and might feel unwanted or inferior. Depending on the circumstance, you might not always feel self-assured. You might, for instance, have a high level of confidence in certain areas, like academics, but a low level of confidence in others, like relationships.

4.1 Self-Confidence vs. Self Esteem

Self-confidence and self-esteem are frequently interchangeable terms. They are, nevertheless, extremely dissimilar. Self-esteem is related to our sense of self and how we interact with the outside world, whereas self-confidence is a measure of our belief in our talents. People frequently go in the wrong direction when these two phrases are confusing, seeking self-esteem through their accomplishments or abilities.

Self-Confidence

The term "self-confidence" refers to our level of assurance in particular life areas. It involves believing in your abilities to accomplish goals and overcome challenges. Self-confidence is externally focused and frequently simpler to develop than self-esteem. The more experience we have with anything, the more confident we get since confidence comes from knowledge and practice. The Latin term fidere, which means "to trust," is where confidence originates. As a result, self-confidence requires believing in oneself and your ability to interact with others. Success experiences frequently result from having self-confidence, which helps that confidence to grow even more. Rather than focusing on improving their self-esteem, most people rely on their self-confidence to be happy.

Self-Esteem

How we feel about ourselves is known as self-esteem and influences our ideas, feelings, and actions. Self-esteem is inward-looking and frequently determines how we interact with the outside environment and other people. Self-esteem, our assessment of our value, derives from the Latin term estimate, which means "to appraise, value, rate, or estimate". Our life experiences and interpersonal relationships help us to develop our self–esteem. Highly self-esteemed people don't need money or status to support themselves and don't worry about failing or getting rejected. They also accept themselves and others as they are, and are open to new experiences in addition to being risk-tolerant.

Is it possible to have self-confidence without self-esteem?

There is no direct link between self-confidence and self-esteem. It's conceivable to have high self-esteem and low self-confidence simultaneously. For instance, a professional athlete or famous person could have high self-confidence in their skills but poor self-esteem and doubt their value. However, having self-confidence in certain aspects of our lives may raise our sense of self-esteem generally, enabling us to work on both at once.

4.2 The Enormous Benefits of Self-Confidence

The advantages of confidence are enormous and can take many forms; they could be social, emotional, mental, and physical. An individual who exudes confidence feels and believes they have plenty to offer, and it pushes them outside of their comfort zone by encouraging them to take chances, explore new opportunities, strive for more in life, overcome obstacles, and accept failure as a necessary step on the road to success. Here are some enormous benefits of self-confidence.

- **You Trust Yourself**

Is there anyone else you should put greater trust in? Trusting in yourself and your skills is a sign of confidence. Having more confidence doesn't mean you have no weaknesses; it just means that you are aware of them and are working to address them. You will have fewer negative thoughts, be able to draw on your past experiences, and know that you can take all possible measures to make things work out. Your strengths are also something you are well aware of and concentrate on.

• Other People Trust You

Teens who are confident radiate trust. Teens who lack self-confidence give the impression to others that they don't trust themselves. People are attracted to self-confident individuals for various reasons, including the power they radiate. People enjoy being around self-confident people. To understand how this principle operates, you must reflect on the "cool kids" from high school.

•Elimination of Self-Doubt

You will defeat your greatest enemy when you gain self-confidence: You. Your deadliest enemies are self-sabotage and self-doubt; therefore, by boosting your confidence, you can turn the script inside your head upside down. As a result, you won't be saying, "*I can't do this,*" but rather, you'll be seizing any chance to learn that comes your way.

• Increased Motivation

You'll discover that you're eager to take on new challenges, learn new skills, and socialize with others. Once you gain self-confidence, you can even surprise yourself with the amount of drive and motivation that you will discover.

• Self-Worth

Self-worth and self-confidence go hand in hand. Due to this, you will begin to appreciate yourself and your opinions once you gain self-confidence.

• **Social Interactions Improve**

In social situations, a lack of confidence can be devastating! In social situations, social anxiety is a severe problem. Social interactions will improve as you gain more self-confidence since those around you will be drawn to your positive vibe. This is how I am, like it or hate it—it's a feeling of self-acceptance! It's empowering and makes it possible to have far more profound social relationships.

• **Confidence Makes You More Physically Attractive**

People with more confidence are more physically appealing. This is because a self-confident person exudes more positive energy and gives off the impression that they are stronger, both of which are desirable traits. You can become more physically beautiful by exuding an aura of confidence that says, *"I know I'm good,"* without actually saying it. Instead of boasting or being overconfident, this is the opposite: confidence in oneself and one's abilities.

4.3 Start Building Social Confidence Today

Are you hiding in the back corner at the party, thinking no one will approach you and engage you in conversation? Recognize that you're not the only one if this describes you. You need to cultivate a confident mindset and work on enhancing your social abilities if you want to become more socially confident. Hopefully, you'll be the one to approach the wallflower at your upcoming party.

Here are some tips to become socially confident:

- **Accept Your Personality**

  Being introverted, or preferring to be alone or with your thoughts, is a trait many people share. If this describes you, don't push yourself to become an extroverted, outgoing person. Anxiety, stress, and even heart problems might result from doing this. Instead, spend time with people you already like and make an effort to engage in meaningful discussion.

- **Understand the Importance of Confidence**

  You can develop social confidence by interacting with others in a way that engages them and makes them feel heard. Social competence combines these abilities and the capacity to elicit genuine listening from others. According to research, developing social skills actually boosts one's positive self-perception and social acceptance.

- **Express Compassion for Others**

  When you deal with other people, you'll foster a positive environment if you show compassion for them. You can increase your confidence by having more fulfilling social encounters. Understanding social cues and empathy are crucial components of interacting meaningfully with others.

- **Maintain Healthy Expectations**

  Even when people try to be social and put themselves forward, they sometimes don't connect. Everyone goes through this; it's natural. To increase your social confidence, keep in mind that you cannot be held accountable for other people's thoughts, feelings, or behaviors.

- **Put Yourself in Social Situations**

Taking advantage of the chance to practice confidence in social settings is crucial. Your social abilities will advance and develop with time, boosting your confidence. Being socially active will also help you feel more at ease, which will eventually help you feel less anxious. Put yourself in various social situations and push yourself to strike up discussions with people.

4.4 Killer Actions to Boost Your Confidence

Humanity depends on having self-confidence. People who are confident in themselves frequently have a positive outlook on life, are satisfied with who they are, and are prepared to take risks to accomplish their objectives. However, a person who lacks self-confidence is less likely to believe that he can accomplish his goals and has a pessimistic outlook on himself and what he expects to achieve in life. The great news is that you can boost your self-confidence totally on your own! Here are some killer actions which will help you boost your confidence:

- *Practicing Self-Care*
To begin boosting your self-confidence, you don't need to look like Brad Pitt. If you want to feel good about who you are and how you appear, take care of yourself by taking daily showers, brushing your teeth, dressing as per your body type, and spending some dedicated time on all aspects of your personality. This doesn't

64

imply that having flashy clothes or a particular style would make you feel more self-assured, but putting an effort to take good care of your appearance sends a message to yourself that you're valuable.

- **Turn Your Negative Thoughts into Positive Ones**

As you become aware of your negative ideas, replace them with positive ones. This could come in the form of encouraging statements like "I'm going to try it, "If I work hard, I can succeed," or "People will pay attention to me." Begin your day with just these few uplifting ideas.

- **Identify Your Talents**

Finding your strengths will help you to concentrate on your talents as everyone has some areas in which they are exceptionally skilled. Permit yourself to feel proud of them. You can express yourself through dance, writing, music, or painting. Find something you like, and then develop a talent that matches it.

- **Accept Compliments Gracefully**

Many individuals with low self-confidence find it difficult to accept compliments because they believe the person is either wrong or lying. You should change how you react to praises if you see yourself rolling your eyes, muttering "Yeah, whatever," or shrugging them off.

- **Stop Comparing Yourself to Others**

If you want to increase your self-confidence, you should concentrate on making your own life better rather than trying to make it more like that of your closest friend, your elder brother, or the superstars you see on the screens. It's important to realize that there will always be people who are prettier, smarter, and wealthier than you, just as there will always be people who are less appealing, less innovative, and maybe less rich than you; all of this is irrelevant; what matters is caring about achieving your dreams and ambitions. Your confidence will increase as a result of this.

- ***Practice Gratitude***

Feelings like you lack anything, whether emotional approval, assets, good fortune, or money, is frequently the basis of uneasiness and lack of confidence. You may fight the sense of being lacking and unsatisfied by recognizing and respecting what you already have. Your spirit will soar once you experience the inner calm that comes with genuine gratitude. Spend some time reflecting on all the positives in your life, such as your lovely friends and your good health.

Chapter 5: Your Activity Toolbox

This chapter will cover some exercises for fostering empathy, enhancing social skills, and boosting self-confidence.

5.1 Activities to Teach Empathy

It's essential to practice waiting, listening, and encouraging the other person to speak without interjecting. It can be cultivated with practice and conscious awareness.

A number of activities have been provided below. Your awareness of the option to listen can be improved with the aid of these activities. Your consciousness and options will increase as you become more conscious of opportunities to switch from talking to listening. They will boost your adaptability and comfort with employing empathy.

Activity 1: Practice with a Partner

Choose a mate. Have your mate talk about anything they want for 90 seconds. You pay attention without speaking. She finishes speaking when the time is up, and you sum up everything she said and any feelings she expressed. When done, talk about the experience. How did it feel for you? How did your partner find it? Change roles and go through the process again.

It might surprise you to learn that you struggle with waiting for the buzzer before speaking. Your determination to resist the impulse to talk may be increased by this realization. Aside from that, agreeing to sum up what you heard would probably make you pay closer attention to the other person's words and body language.

Activity 2: Exercise in Self-Awareness and Choice

When you're listening the next time and feel like talking about something you're interested in but the other person hasn't paused, keep listening. Wait two to three seconds if the other has stopped. If she or he starts speaking again, pay attention. Talk if she doesn't start up again.

Waiting is necessary because the talker can be taking a break to collect her thoughts before speaking again.

Activity 3: Practice Listening & Summarizing

When the speaker pauses for longer than three or four seconds and you are prepared to discuss your interests, sum up instead. Continue listening if they start chatting again. Talk if they don't start back up. Knowing that you comprehended what she was saying can inspire the speaker to speak further. Alternatively, she might delay if she's unsure of your wants to learn more but is hesitant to inquire. However, if you sum up her points rather than expressing your own interests, she could assume that you want to listen more. Of course, summarizing is recognizing the talker's words, not his emotions. Summarizing what has been said is adequate for this task. It facilitates the exercise and adds value.

Activity 4: Pace of Practice

Exercise at a pace that seems appropriate to you. Practice exercise #2, for instance, for two to three minutes every day for a week. Then, for the following week or two, extend your daily time to five to ten minutes. Increase the frequency of this exercise gradually, up to the point where you can bear to briefly shut off thought or conversation about your interests.

5.2 Activities to Build Confidence in Teens

Here are five activities to increase your self-assurance that not only will do so but also help you feel better about yourself, making them excellent instruments for self-improvement and empowerment:

Activity 1: Focus on Improving Your Strengths Rather Than Your Weaknesses

When things aren't going your way, it is quite simple to get down and concentrate on your flaws. A typical emotion known as negativity bias causes you to focus on the negative rather than the positive. Therefore, rather than rectifying your weaknesses during challenging times, it is a terrific confidence-building activity to concentrate on and work on your strengths. If you're having a bad day, sit down with a piece of paper and a pen and list three things you appreciate about yourself and three things you're good at. Improve those areas of strength, and you'll see an increase in your confidence.

Activity 2: Honor Every Victory, No Matter How Small or Great

You endured seven days of successful exercise? Give yourself a high five. *Completed a significant assignment prior to the due date?* Go out to a nice supper for yourself. *Successfully resolved a friend's issue?* Watch television while sipping coffee. When you give yourself a reward for completing a task, you're training your brain to release the feel-good hormone dopamine. This can help you to maintain your motivation and happiness while directly boosting your confidence levels.

Activity 3: Meditation and Mindfulness Exercises

One of the most potent and effective ways to gain confidence is through regular meditation practice. It improves your mindset, provides you time to ponder, analyzes your thoughts, and enables you to connect with your deepest thoughts and feelings. Meditation can help you become happier, more confident, and better at making decisions over time.

5.3 Social Skills Activities for Teens

When we have social anxiety, we may avoid social situations, which might have an impact on how we develop connections. Teens who struggle with social anxiety often have a strong fear of public speaking, which can have a bad effect. Teens with anxiety, a fear of public speaking, and other comparable challenges can achieve their best functioning by participating in social skill-building activities.

Here are some social skills building activities.

Activity 1: Dining Out

Dining with friends is something that almost everyone on the earth appreciates, especially when trying out new or intriguing foods. Eating can be one of life's greatest pleasures because everyone needs to eat. To keep things interesting, make an effort to frequently try new restaurants and invite your friends or others you would like to know better, to lunch or dinner.

Activity 2: Movie Nights

Invite your neighbors and friends over to your house to watch movies. You will be able to chat, rewind, and query others. Get comfortable being a social snoop to learn what genres they enjoy and why. Practice your small talk so you can have a conversation about the movie and find points of agreement.

Activity 3: Volunteering

While learning small chat, collaborating with others, and hopefully building connections and friends, you may contribute to making the world a better place. Better still, think of organizing a charity walk or run or a beach clean-up day; having a purpose provides us an excuse to help others.

A Conclusive Checklist for Self Evaluation

A group of learned social behaviors and abilities known as social skills, or empathy, are often displayed in interpersonal settings. Developing social skills will enable you to work with others to solve problems in an organized and efficient manner.

To attain the best possible social outcomes and deeper connections, it is crucial to cultivate social skills and empathy within oneself. Accordingly, effective application of social skills and empathy is advantageous for

- *Becoming more expressive.*
- *Being aware of other's emotions*
- *Making sure others don't stop you from attaining your goals.*

Additionally,

- *It enables you to interact with people accurately, effectively, and amicably.*
- *Adequately and confidently express your feelings, desires, ideas, or rights.*
- *Take into consideration everyone's interests and needs.*
- *When an issue arises, try to find the most reasonable solution for everyone.*

Not everyone finds it simple to go out and socialize with others. Some people are concerned about embarrassing themselves in front of others and becoming a laughingstock. However, others think they don't belong elsewhere because they don't seem to fit in with others. These people might be having a difficult time managing their social lives for a variety of reasons.

72

If you fall into this category, it's time to discard this false notion. Nothing is wrong with you. You have the same qualities as everyone else, including potential and weaknesses. You share the same traits as everyone else. It's time to free yourself from the demons that have long been enslaving your senses and existed only in your thoughts. If you don't want to live in pain for the rest of your life, it's time to realize your full potential. Humans are sociable beings by nature. We have to interact with others from the time we are born until the day we die away, whether they are friends, family, or total strangers we meet on the street.

Relationships and connections that go well between people can develop into friendships. Without others' help, it is difficult to advance in life; thus, building strong interpersonal relationships is important. You may increase your self-confidence by reducing the negative effects of stress and by developing more and stronger relationships.

SOCIAL SKILLS SELF-CHECKLISTS

Which skills do you believe require improvement? Place a checkmark next to the sentence that seems to be true for you.

_____ I struggle to comprehend other people's thoughts and emotions.

_____ I struggle to get along with others.

_____ I can't maintain friendships for very long.

_____ When I'm being spoken to, I easily become distracted.

_____I shy away from the conversation because I don't know what to say.

_____My jokes typically don't elicit laughter from others.

_____I'm pretty susceptible to peer pressure.

_____I have trouble reading the body language and facial expressions of other individuals.

_____I occasionally say inappropriate things.

_____I lack the conversational skills to keep a conversation going.

_____I have anxiety and nervousness around individuals.

Where Do I Need to "Grow" and Where am I a "Pro"?

Depending on how proficient you believe you are at each skill, mark it as **"Pro"** or "**Grow**."

Empathy Related Skill	Pro	Grow
1. Compromising		
2. Obeying instructions		
3. Showing Empathy		
4. Sharing		
5. Apologizing		
6. Expressing Emotions		
7. Accepting Consequences		
8. Flexible Thinking		
9. Disagreeing Respectfully		
10. Using self-control		
11. Respecting personal space		

If you are a pro at anything, highlight the word in green; if you need to grow, underline the word in yellow.

Printed in Great Britain
by Amazon

36942153R00046